Contents

CW00705303

Author's note: Some hospitals provide information to patients, before admission. This is by no means universal and sometimes inadequate. This booklet offers practical tips and easy-to-follow advice for anyone who is about to be admitted to hospital.

Sources: The source of all facts and figures is Office of National Statistics, National Institute for Health and Clinical Guidance, and Chairman of Parliamentary Thrombosis Group.

Introduction

In the United Kingdom, we are very fortunate to have the National Health Service in which I have had the privilege of serving for over forty years.

Recently, I found myself at the receiving end as a patient requiring hospital treatment. It was during this period that it occurred to me that all fellow patients should be aware of a few avoidable pitfalls of hospitalisation, as their life could depend on it.

Most of us will have to be admitted to hospital one day. When the time comes, you are most grateful that hospitals exist where professionals will take care of you, relieve your suffering and hopefully bring you back to your normal self.

It is true that you lose some control of your daily life in hospital. With your hope of full recovery comes a slight fear that you may not survive or that the experience will be unpleasant, embarrassing or painful. Most fears are unfounded and come out of misconceptions. There is plenty you can do to help yourself and take responsibility for your own health.

Being informed and confident will give you the best chance of a speedy recovery.

Before you go into hospital

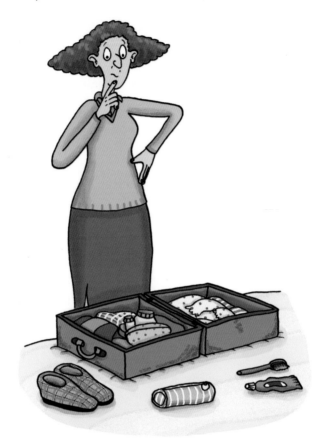

"There are plenty of things you may
need in hospital."

The will to survive

It is very rare for anyone to die on the operating table these days. Anaesthesia is very safe. The advances in medicine and technology have given doctors the skills to deal with unexpected events, which, at one time, might have proved fatal.

Trust the professionals

We have learnt more in the last fifty years than the previous two thousand years. Trust the professionals and their judgment; feel safe in the knowledge that they will do everything they can to help you to recover.

Think positively

Have a positive attitude and the will to survive any illness, no matter how low you feel. Think of your family and friends who want you to live and to share with them the joys that life has to offer. Remember the pleasure it gives you to see a smile on a child's face and to receive a hug from a loved one. Be determined to witness the colours of next spring, the sunshine of the summer, the glorious scenery in the autumn and festivities of Christmas or other special days.

If you have grandchildren, they will give you the inspiration to fight and survive your illness; you will want to see them grow up into beautiful people. Don't underestimate the benefits of owning a pet; their unconditional love and your responsibility for its wellbeing will also give you a reason to survive.

Plan for the future

If possible, before going into hospital, invest in the future by planting bulbs, flowers, shrubs and especially climbers as you can witness their growth and progress daily during your recovery. Ask your doctor when you are likely to be able to travel after your admission or operation; it is worth considering booking a holiday in advance. This will be something to look forward to; relaxing somewhere in the sun would help your recovery and lift your spirits.

Continue to buy lottery tickets if this is what you already do.

We are living longer

Throughout the world people are living longer. In the United Kingdom, we are fortunate to have an excellent chance of living a long life. According to UK Government statistics, an average man can expect to live up to 79.5 years and a woman to 82.5 years.

At present, medicine and surgery are undergoing a period of revolution. Many conditions which until comparatively recently were considered inoperable or untreatable, are now being successfully managed and cured. Diagnosis can be made early, thanks to advanced imaging and scanning.

There are constant developments in transplant surgery, immunology, genetics, technology and microsurgery, leading to some doctors predicting possible cures for various cancers, cardiovascular disease and dementia, making us more optimistic and confident about our future life.

Lifespan and realism

We all have to die someday. Major illnesses such as cancer, heart disease, stroke, diabetes and Alzheimer's disease are a reality and as you get older, your chances of contracting one or more of these diseases increase. Be realistic and prepare for the future and your peace of mind.

Before going into hospital, think about the following:

- Seek legal advice and **make sure you have made your will**. We should all have made a will, regardless of our health.

- **Sort out your accounts** and get advice from the bank manager or accountant.

- If at all possible, **involve your spouse/partner** in these matters. No one should be totally ignorant of their finances, assets, debts and their mortgage situation.

- **Talk to your family and friends** and let them know when you are going into hospital. They will want to help in any way they can, wish you good luck and may feel left out if they are not informed.

- **Build yourself up.** You are going to need all your reserves. Watch your diet and eat healthily. Take reasonable exercise daily. Even if you have only a few days before you are admitted, it will help you enormously to exercise, expand your lungs, mobilise your joints and get your circulation going. If you are overweight, try to lose a little. It is never too late to start.

- If you smoke, **quit smoking.** This might be the single best thing you can do for yourself. It will help recovery after surgery; reduce potential coughing which would subsequently reduce the strain and pain of stitches being pulled. It will diminish your chances of clot formation in the legs and pelvic veins. It will accelerate healing of your wound. It will reduce your chances of having a heart attack or a stroke and lower your blood pressure.

- **Tidy up the garden**, if possible. When you return home, you may not be able to cut the grass or do heavy work for a while. It is always pleasing to admire a tidy garden. Plant a shrub, preferably one which is covered in buds and water it thoroughly. You will appreciate the blooms during your period of recovery.

- Ask someone to water your plants (indoors and outdoors) while you are away, as well as collect your mail.

- Cancel the newspapers.

- Arrange care for your pet.

- Turn the central heating down.

- Make sure your home is secure.

What to pack

There are plenty of things you may need in hospital. Here are about 30 suggestions:

- **List of telephone numbers** to contact people.

- **Notepad/pencil** to make notes, write down names and questions.

- **Book/magazine/newspaper.**

- **Glasses/contact lenses/hearing aids.**

- **Keys** for your home when you return.

- **Mobile phone:** There are certain areas in hospitals where phones cannot be used. It can interrupt a conversation with a doctor or nurse and it can be annoying for other patients who may be resting. It is useful when you need it and personal patient line calls are expensive, so keep your phone in a silent mode and use text messaging, which is unlikely to disturb anyone.

- **List of medications.** Do not take your stock of prescribed pills with you. They will probably be confiscated and some hospitals have a policy to allow patients to take medication, which has only been dispensed by their own pharmacies. They will discharge you on a meagre supply and you may have to contact your own doctor's surgery for a fresh prescription as soon as you are discharged.

- Minimum **two or three nighties or pairs of pyjamas.** You are going to wear these all the time in a heated and dry environment and there is more likelihood of soiling your clothes with food, drink, perspiration or other bodily fluids than in normal circumstances. Whenever possible, a daily change of clothes after a shower or bath should be the aim as you would in your normal life. Perhaps a relative or friend can wash and change them for you on a regular basis.

- **Dressing gown.** A lightweight gown (washable cotton is preferable) will help to protect your dignity. Most hospital gowns tie at the back and leave your posterior exposed as you get in and out of bed.

- **Slippers** (disposable!). Use them in hospital and dispose of them when you are discharged. You do not want to bring hospital bugs back home.
- **Electric toothbrush.** When you are really ill or weak or after an abdominal or chest operation it can be uncomfortable to use your forearm and wrist to brush your teeth. An electric toothbrush is effortless and thorough. For those with dentures, a container and cleaning tablets will be useful.
- **An electric shaver** for men is convenient.
- **Alcohol-based gel** (available from chemists) to keep hands clean.
- **Perfume, aftershave/deodorant**: recommended for your morale and creating a pleasant atmosphere around you when your personal space will be invaded several times by so many.
- **Long-handled shower brush.** It is essential to keep ultra clean, especially in hospital when your natural resistance to infections is low. A long handle will help you to scrub areas of your body, which you might otherwise neglect.
- **Petroleum jelly (for example, Vaseline) or lip balm.** The dry atmosphere will tend to dry your lips and nostrils. Often you may not be allowed drinks orally. Applying petroleum jelly to your lips and nostrils will make a difference.
- **Nasal spray or inhaler** (for example, Vicks). In the immediate post-operative period it may be uncomfortable even to blow your nose. A nasal spray may offer temporary relief and help you to breathe through your nose.
- **Cold sore cream** (for example, Zovirax containing acyclovir). Millions of people get cold sores and are prone to developing them when their

resistance is low. To avoid this, start applying cream at the first sign of burning sensation on the lip.

- **Small packets of tissues** are likely to come in handy. Avoid large boxes, which are exposed to the hospital air for days.

- **Soft toilet paper.** Some hospitals have poor quality toilet paper. Remember it is your responsibility to keep yourself as clean and hygienic as you possibly can.

- **Moist toilet tissues.** Easier to use and help with further cleanliness. Wet wipes. For frequent cleaning of hands or face.

- **Fresh air spray.** When you first open your bowels after a major operation or an acute illness, it will not always be easy. You are likely to need a commode and likely to be separated from other patients only by curtains. It will be kinder to others if you use the spray as well as turning on your radio!

  Note: Some hospitals discourage the use of aerosol sprays or perfumes, in case of allergic reactions in other patients.

- **A rolled-up taped towel.** This is an essential piece of "equipment" you need to take with you. Roll up a towel into the shape and size of a loaf of bread and secure the ends with tape so that it does not unroll. Its use is described later on page 17.

- **200ml drinks with straw,** small chocolate bars, biscuits, small assorted cereal packets, food and drink that can be consumed as a snack and not stored after opening the packaging.

- **Personal items** such as a face cloth and mirror.

- **Radio, CD player**...useful personal entertainment.

- **Headphones** for personal entertainment or noise exclusion.

- **Electric socket adaptor** and chargers.

- **Money** for newspapers or the television.

- **Eye mask**. To cut out the glaring lights at night in the ward to allow you to achieve your much-needed sleep.

- **Ear plugs**. Invaluable to cut out the clangs and bangs allowing you to sleep. The wards can be busy and noisy during the night with new admissions and squeaky trolleys.

- **Liquid soap**, shampoo, conditioner and shower cap. Nail clippers.

- **Mints**.

- Consider packing everything in a small bag on wheels

  Note: Do not take any expensive items such as watches and jewellery with you into hospital.

Recommendations before admission

- Cut toenails. Remember to wash between your toes. You do not know when you'll reach them again comfortably! Cut all nails as they may harbour germs. Have a haircut. Bath/shave and shampoo your hair before you go into hospital.

- Prepare a few meals and freeze them.

- If you are due for an operation start using medicated soap such as a chlorhexidine-based soap or povidine iodine liquid soap for three days prior to your admission. This will reduce the bacterial flora normally resident in your skin.

- Tell your close family and friends truthfully about the diagnosis and your treatment. They would prefer to hear it from you and would want to support you. Children may need reassurance and explanations as to how your illness might affect them.

While you are in hospital

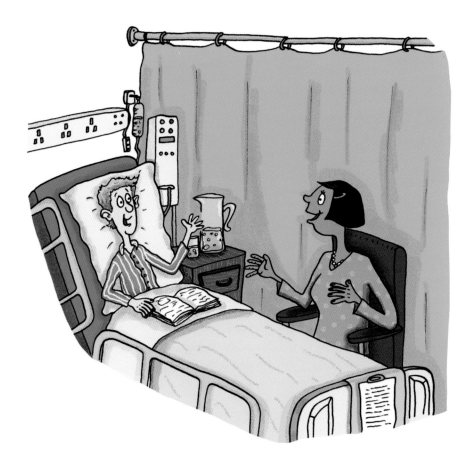

"Most patients enjoy visits from their loved ones."

The real risks of hospitalisation

No matter what the reason is for your admission, as a hospital in-patient you are at risk of several common conditions, which can be debilitating and sometimes fatal. These are often preventable and you should be aware of the potential dangers so you can try to reduce the risk of getting them.

You can do much to help yourself by reducing the risk of the following conditions:

- Deep Vein Thrombosis (DVT)

- Chest infection

- Hospital-acquired infections (MRSA and Clostridium difficilis)

- Dehydration

- Urinary tract infection

- Wind and constipation

- Pain

Deep Vein Thrombosis (DVT)

Hospital-acquired DVT is the most common cause of hospital mortality. Deep vein thrombosis can lead to pulmonary embolus (a clot migrating to the lung), which can be fatal. At least two thirds of deaths are preventable.

Over 50 per cent of all hospital patients are at risk of developing DVT and, in the UK, every year about 100,000 hospital patients develop DVT, out of which over 25,000 die due to pulmonary embolism.

About 60 per cent of our body is composed of water in the form of tissue fluid, various secretions, lymph and blood. The fluid is in constant motion and circulated mainly by the pumping action of the heart. During admission to hospital when we lie still for hours, the circulation slows down and in some areas it almost comes to a standstill. This makes us prone to thrombosis, particularly in the calf and pelvic veins (the same risk applies on aeroplane flights lasting over four hours).

Conditions involving slow circulation, vessel wall injury and increased tendency to clotting of blood or involving reduced mobility for three days can lead to DVT.

Who is more at risk?

Smokers, obese people, diabetics, those on HRT (hormone replacement therapy) or the oral contraceptive pill, those with a previous or family history of thrombosis and those who are over 50 years old are more at risk.

Some surgical procedures carry a much higher risk of DVT, such as operations on the lower limbs (up to 70 per cent risk after hip or knee replacements), major abdominal and pelvic or gynaecological operations (25-30 per cent risk).

40-50 per cent of patients admitted with a stroke or heart attack are at risk of DVT. Cancer patients have three times more chance of DVT than non-cancer patients. Fractures and trauma increase risk of DVT considerably.

This is preventable and you should be proactive to protect yourself.

What can you do?

- Quit smoking no matter how long you have had the habit. There might be immediate benefits.

- Discuss with your GP whether to continue with the oral contraceptive pill or HRT whilst you are in hospital.

- Lose weight if you need to and take exercise.

- Avoid alcohol for at least two days before surgery and keep hydrated – at least half a glass an hour.

- Discuss with your surgeon about the use of graduated compression bandage or surgical stockings (the same are advertised for use during long haul flights).

Keep moving

Try and exercise different parts of your body when you are confined to bed in a hospital.

As soon as you wake up from anaesthesia, wriggle your toes, move your fingers, wrists, ankles and any part of your body that does not hurt. Get your circulation going; the nurses and physiotherapists can't do it for you.

Do not lie still during your waking hours. Use the buttons on the control panel to raise the foot end of the bed from time to time so that your feet are at a higher level than your pelvis to help drain blood from your legs.

Gently exercise your toes and ankles in bed. By moving your foot up and down you use your calf muscles as pumps to circulate blood.

In some hospitals anti-coagulants are used during and after the surgery to prevent clots (DVT). Some hospitals use graduated elastic stockings or intermittent pneumatic compression devices on legs to prevent DVT.

Chest infection and pneumonia

After abdominal surgery, about 20 per cent of patients have some degree of chest infection. After surgery the breathing is mostly shallow and the lungs do not have the opportunity to expand fully. With gravity the secretions tend to go to the back and the base of the lungs.

Plugs of mucus can block small bronchi and lead to a collapse of segments of lung tissue, which leads to infection.

Because it hurts to cough after most chest and abdominal operations, the normal urge to cough is voluntarily suppressed, increasing the risk of chest infection by retaining mucous or phlegm.

Who is more at risk?

Admission in a medical ward for a stroke, heart, kidney or renal failure, which necessitates prolonged bed rest, can make you vulnerable to chest infection. The longer you lie flat, the higher your risk of chest infection.

The very young and the very old are vulnerable. Smokers, the obese and pregnant patients are a high risk. Patients taking steroids or who are immunologically compromised are vulnerable. It applies to all patients who are immobile.

What can you do?

Quit smoking.

If you have an existing chest infection, get it treated before admission to hospital. Some doctors may prescribe antibiotics as a precaution.

If you are over 60 or vulnerable to chest infections, have your yearly flu jab.

If at all possible, try to arrange surgery during a time of year when your chest is usually better. Practise deep breathing and holding your breath for three seconds, several times a day.

Anyone who comes to visit you and has a cold or cough should stay at least six feet away. Ask the ward staff to provide them with a disposable face mask.

Breathing exercises

As soon as you wake up from the anaesthetic, take a few deep breaths.

As you get confident, expand your lungs fully and hold for three seconds before breathing out. Take another deep breath, hold it for three seconds and breathe in some more air and again hold. Finally, you will be able to inhale and hold a bit more air the third time before exhaling. Repeat 5-10 times an hour.

The lungs are like balloons. When you breathe in, their elasticity lets them expand to accommodate the air and after a while when they get used to the stretching, they can accept more air and expand further. We rarely use them to their full capacity.

Similarly breathe out and hold for three seconds. Try to breathe out some more, then hold; finally you will be surprised that the third time you can exhale further before breathing normally. In this way, you are trying to expand and contract your lungs as much as you comfortably can, preventing infections.

Cough it up

If you feel that there is a plug of mucus in your chest, you must cough it up. Before attempting to cough, sit up. You may have an electric bed or ask a nurse to help. Next, have a sip of water. It is easier to move the plug of thick mucus while sitting up if you have lubricated your throat.

Now, before you cough, blow out short sharp puffs of air with your mouth open, as if moistening your lenses with your breath before cleaning your glasses. This, surprisingly, will not hurt, unlike coughing, which surely would after an abdominal or chest operation. When you feel that the mucus is within range in the throat, place the rolled-up towel (see What to pack on page 10) on top of your wound and press with your forearm and with the other hand catch the mucus in a tissue over your mouth as you give a mighty cough. You have to win the battle of the airways!

Chest infection or pneumonia on top of your existing illness will delay your recovery and prolong your stay in hospital.

Note: Some of these rules may not apply after eye, ear or brain surgery. Talk to the professionals concerned with your case.

Hospital-acquired infections

In the UK, since 2007 the number of deaths linked with hospital-acquired deaths has dropped significantly, Many of us are un-necessarily worried about super bugs. They do exist however, and Clostridium difficile claims about 1600 lives and MRSA is involved in under 300 deaths. These figures are reducing every year due to better awareness and improved hygiene in hospitals. The infections vary from hospital to hospital and depend on the type of operation, overcrowding and the length of stay. All surgeons know their infection rates, should you want to ask!

Clostridium difficile and MRSA (Methicillin-resistant Staphylococcus aureus) are two of the common hospital bugs. It is worth knowing a little about them. Hospitals admit patients with all sorts of infections, which can at times be difficult to eradicate completely from the environment.

Clostridium difficile is spread by faecal contamination of food or water and leads to diarrhoea in vulnerable patients, especially those who have received antibiotics for other infections. Their spores can live in the environment for a long time. Strict personal hygiene of patients, staff in hospitals, clean kitchens, wards and toilets are of paramount importance.

Hospital patients who develop MRSA can expect their length of stay to triple. This bacterium is spread by direct contact and usually causes wound infection. It can be resistant to most antibiotics and patients will be isolated to prevent further spread. These bacteria can live in the nostrils without showing any signs or symptoms. Nasal swabs can identify MRSA carriers and antibiotic nasal creams can help to prevent the spread of this infection. Some MRSA produce an enzyme called leucocidin, a potent toxin, which kills white blood cells.

In addition to Clostridium Difficile and MRSA, there is Stenotrophomonas maltophilia (Steno), which thrives in the black muck that can surround shower-heads and taps. It is responsible for about 300 deaths per year in the UK. There is also an increase in the incidence of infections caused by MSSA (a variant of MRSA) and Glyco-peptide resistant enterococci (GRE).

Hospitals have introduced protocols to reduce infections, improved staff awareness and raised standards of cleanliness.

Who is more at risk?

- All immuno-compromised patients
- Diabetics
- Patients on steroids
- Smokers
- Chronically ill patients
- People with poor personal hygiene.

What can you do?

Three to five days before admission, a daily shower using chlorhexidine or povidine iodine soap (available from chemists), will help to reduce skin bacterial flora.

Cut your nails prior to admission. Wash your hands before you touch food.

When you wake up from anaesthesia, shift the position of your bottom and roll your body as often as you can comfortably, so that you do not apply constant pressure to one area of skin causing possible damage.

Make sure that the sheets are not creased or wet. If wet in the slightest, get them changed. While in the hospital, avoid touching your mouth or nose with your hands and avoid resting food on furniture or bed linen.

When you go to the toilet, whenever possible use some paper or disposable tissues as a barrier before you touch door handles, use taps, pull cords or touch the toilet flush handle. Let the water run in the shower for a short while before you use it.

Be observant. Make sure that nurses and doctors wash their hands before examining you. Wash your own hands regularly and ask visitors to do the same. Unwell relatives should not visit you or if in doubt, ask for a disposable mask for them. There are alcohol-based dispensers in each ward for hand washing. They are effective but do not replace proper hand washing with soap to prevent Clostridium difficile spread.

If your intravenous drip site feels wet, let the nurse know. If your wound dressing is wet or soiled get it changed. If your drain, catheter or tubes are wet, they need attention.

Nurses will encourage you to get out of bed the day after the operation. This is good for you even for a short time. This helps to prevent DVT, helps with breathing and encourages burping.

If you need to use a bedpan, make sure you wipe yourself as best as you can. Use moist toilet tissue. Ask for a bowl of water if necessary. Dry yourself thoroughly. The cleanliness of your perineum (area between your pubis and your coccyx or tail bone) is your responsibility. Do not forget the deodorant spray!

If you can walk to the toilet, you may find reaching your perineum a difficult task after an operation. Sitting on the front edge of the toilet seat, on one buttock may give you easier access to clean yourself. Always wash your hands thoroughly afterwards.

Do not be afraid to ask questions. If you are worried about being too assertive, just remember your life could be at stake.

A good idea! If you think someone is going to examine you who may not have washed their hands, apply a blob of alcohol gel on your right palm and offer to shake their hand transferring the gel and apologising for your 'carelessness'!

Doctors and nurses should wash their hands and wipe the diaphragm of their stethoscopes before touching any patient. Disposable gloves should be used wherever possible.

All patients should remain vigilant and protect themselves against possible infections.

Quit smoking. Smokers are three times more likely to get infections, have slow wound healing and a longer stay in hospital.

Control your diabetes before admission, as there is more likelihood of acquired infection.

Dehydration

In the dry atmosphere and usually overheated hospital wards, it is easy to get dehydrated. Remember to have adequate water to drink. Most adults require two litres per day in average conditions. Thirst and a dry mouth are reliable signs that you need more fluids.

Who is more at risk?

If you are running a high temperature, perspiring, losing blood or suffering from diarrhoea, you may be at further risk of dehydration.

What can you do?

Drink plenty of fluids. Make sure that your jug of water is covered with a lid to keep the water clean. Bottled water or 200 ml drink cartons of your favourite fruit juice are worth considering.

If you are on an intravenous drip and the fluid in the bottle runs out, do not hesitate to draw the attention of a nurse.

Urinary Tract Infections

It may surprise you to know that urinary tract infection is the most common hospital-acquired infection, accounting for 40 per cent of all hospital-acquired infections.

Who is more at risk?

The main cause of this infection is the prolonged use of an indwelling catheter. The risk of urinary tract infection increases dramatically if the catheter is retained for more than six days.

What can you do?

If you have a catheter, ask the doctor every day if you still need it. Hospital doctors have a lot to remember and they might forget you still have a catheter inside you.

Adequate fluid intake and adequate urinary output will help to prevent urinary infection. Drink plenty of fluids and maintain good hygiene, especially in the genital area by regular washing with soap and water.

If there is the slightest burning or discomfort at the site where the catheter enters your body, tell the nurse or the doctor.

Antimicrobial, suprapubic and condom type catheters are known to reduce the risk of infection.

Wind and constipation

You may notice that your abdomen swells up like a balloon a day or two after the operation or after the nasal tube has been removed. This is usually wind collected in the stomach and will easily come up if you attempt to get out of bed to sit in a chair, with help if required.

Who is more at risk?

With the inevitable lack of exercise, reduced food intake and use of painkillers, constipation can be a problem.

What can you do?

Ask for professional help if you are uncomfortable. Do not be embarrassed. Cereals, wholewheat bread, fruit and vegetables will help.

Pain

This does not have to be a problem. Ask for help if you are uncomfortable. Do not test your pain threshold and let the pain establish. Pain can demoralise you and delay your recovery. If you are connected to a morphine pump, use it. You cannot overdose yourself as it has a failsafe mechanism.

If you have had abdominal keyhole surgery, pain around the shoulders is common in the first 24 to 48 hours.

Catheter and drains

When you visit someone in a hospital and notice intra-venous drips, abdominal/chest drains and urinary catheter attached to them, it can be a frightening sight and you may cringe at the thought of having the same experience. These are surprisingly easy to tolerate and you are usually not aware of their presence. You are likely to be pleasantly surprised by the lack of discomfort and the ease with which they are removed.

Shower/Bath

It is your responsibility to keep clean. No one will tell you to shower or change your clothes daily. In your daily life you shower or have a bath and change your clothes at least once. It is essential to keep clean and stay hygienic even more when you are not well. Change your clothes at least once a day. Ask the nursing staff for help if you need it.

The bathrooms in the hospital are well equipped to assist you with extra grab rails, bath seats and high toilet seats. There is always a good supply of towels. A long-handled brush, face cloth and liquid soap are useful.

Ask for help, if you need it, to get in or out of the bath. It usually does not matter if your wound or dressing gets wet in the shower, though it will need changing soon afterwards. It is a good idea to ask the nurses if you can go for a shower, as they will be better prepared to change your dressings afterwards.

Notepad and pencil

Note down the names of the anaesthetist, surgical team, physicians, nurses, physiotherapists, pharmacists, radiographers, auxiliary staff porters and administrators you come into contact with.

Visitors

Ask your family to appoint one person who will ring the ward to check on your progress and cascade the information to others. This will avoid repetitive enquiry about the same patient and free ward staff for other duties.

Most patients enjoy visits from their loved ones. Grandchildren are a special joy. Gifts, cards, magazines and chocolates are all welcome and cheering. If the hospital allows them, flowers or a small plant are always welcome (except in chest departments). Baskets of fruit attract germs and dust so ask relatives to bring a manageable portion of fruit salad, in a sealed plastic box, and a disposable sealed spoon/fork. Daily fresh fruit is good for you. Try having fruit salad twice a day! Ice cream is easy to digest too.

As you gain strength and gradually get mobile in hospital, observe if there are any fellow patients who have not received visitors. It might be a good idea to pay them a brief visit for a chat to cheer them up!

When you come out of hospital

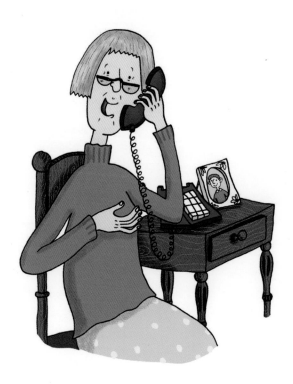

"Take the first step, call your friends to
put them at their ease."

Returning home

- Write thank you letters or cards to the anaesthetist, your surgical team, the ward staff and everybody who was kind to you. Mention them by name. They have received enough criticism in the past and a thank you letter is a precious reward for them and would be most welcome.

- Your bed at home is likely to be lower than the hospital bed and it may be harder to get up without help. You may need a table or a chair next to your bed for support in getting up. A backrest and extra pillows may be helpful.

- Men may find a urine bottle helpful for a few days before they can manage to get out of bed unassisted. Ask for one or two disposable ones from the ward staff before you leave the hospital. It will be especially useful at night, as you may not have to disturb anyone else for help in getting up.

- It is also useful to have a bath seat or a plastic chair or stool in the bath on which to sit down and a sturdy chair near the toilet to help you when getting up.

- You will finally need help with your socks/tights/stockings and shoes. Once you can manage those, you have more than likely recovered and gained your strength. If you find it hard to dry the skin between your toes, try pulling a sock or towel up and down in between your toes before putting it on.

- Your recovery may be slower than you expect. Be patient and remember that your body will need time to get back to your original state of fitness.

Communicating with friends

You may notice a change in the attitude of your friends towards you when you return home. Take the initiative and talk to your friends by phone or email to tell them that you are back home. Some may be hesitant to contact you, not knowing how you feel. Others may think they might be disturbing you and your recovery. Some find it very difficult to resume ordinary friendships or even conversation after you have been diagnosed with a serious illness such as cancer. Some of your friends may be worried about breaking down and crying in front of you. They are afraid to say the wrong thing or sometimes what to say to you at all!

Take the first step instead and call them to put them at their ease. When my friends asked what they could do for me? I always replied, "lend us a fiver". This broke the ice and created a good laugh. Only one of them actually gave me a fiver (which I accepted!).

Many of your close friends genuinely want to help you and be useful. Try and accept the offer they make as it is beneficial for both of you and strengthens the bond between you. If you delay or lose contact with your friends, you may feel unsupported and isolated.

Most friends will ask, "is there anything at all I can do?". Try and say, "yes, please."

Depending on their talents and your mood, you could suggest that they:

- Take you for a drive

- Read to you

- Play indoor games with you

- Find a DVD or a book that you always wanted

- Accompany you to the hospital, or the pharmacist

- Mow the lawn

- Take on the D.I.Y. job you had planned

- Do the shopping for you

- Help to plan a pleasant surprise for your family/carer

- Give you company and your carer a short break.

Reactions of people you meet after your illness

Be prepared for several tactless or unhelpful remarks as they are uttered spontaneously when you meet people whom you have not seen for some time. They can give you a look of surprise as if seeing someone they had not expected to be mobile or even alive. Having once been labelled as seriously ill, they may have mentally written you off.   Reassure them with smile or a quip.

Most of your friends and acquaintances will be genuinely glad to see you and remark that you look well and have the sparkle back in your eyes. Some will not believe you when you tell them that you are really better. They will double check with your spouse and want to know the truth.

Thank the hospital staff

You may feel it appropriate to give something to the nurses and other members of the staff in the wards who were kind to you, looked after you and made your stay as comfortable as possible. Consider gifts that can be shared, for example:

- Box of chocolates or biscuits

- Supplies of tea/coffee and sugar

- Crockery (coffee mugs or tea cups and saucers)

- Vouchers from supermarkets (useful for ward parties)

- A painting.

If in doubt, telephone and ask someone on the ward.

- A bottle of wine for your consultant. Phone the consultant's secretary and ask about his/her favourite tipple!

- A thank you letter or even a gift for your GP if you feel that he or she was helpful, kind and prompt in diagnosing your ailment and referring you to the hospital.

Your spouse/partner/carer

Spare a thought for them. It is a good idea to buy a thank you present or flowers for your carer telling them frequently how much you love and appreciate them. It is often forgotten that if someone is ill, the whole family suffers. This is a very stressful time for your carer and their whole life revolves around you and your welfare.

Driving

You will know when you are fit to drive safely and without discomfort. Do not drive if your medication makes you feel drowsy or dizzy. You should be able to make an emergency stop. Try applying brakes in your stationary car and see if it causes any discomfort. If in doubt, ask your doctor about your fitness to drive.

In the UK, it is illegal to drive within 48 hours after having a general anaesthetic. It is also your responsibility to inform the DVLA and your car insurance company if you have had a serious illness, which may affect your driving.

Christmas, New Year, and other special occasions

There are old friends and acquaintances with whom you communicate once a year by sending a greetings card. Don't be too surprised if they telephone you unexpectedly before sending their card to make sure that you are still alive!

The Future

Be well informed and ask questions about how best to maintain good health in the future. Watching your weight, eating healthily and drinking in moderation are habits to nurture. Take regular exercise. Protect yourself from prolonged exposure to sunlight.

If you are unfortunate and experience unusual symptoms or notice any unexpected changes in your body, seek medical advice at an early stage.

Do not ignore new or changing moles on your skin or a lump in the breast or testicles. Any unexpected bleeding or a change in your bowel habit should be reported to your doctor. If you have a persistent cough or a hoarse voice for three weeks, seek medical advice.

Remember that an early diagnosis will always give you a better chance of survival and uncomplicated recovery. There is always hope, no matter how serious the condition. It is essential to take responsibility for your own health.

Good health is rarely appreciated until it is lost!

My best wishes,

Rami Seth

Dr Rami Seth MBE FRCS

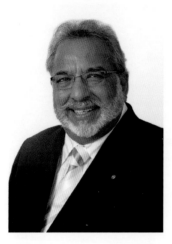

"After my operation, when I woke up in the intensive care unit in St. James's Hospital in Leeds, I could only see the top of my dressing, as I was lying flat. I asked the nurse how far down my scar went. She bent down and whispered in my ear, "from tits to the tail, love, and a bit on the side." I immediately had a good belly laugh and understood her precise anatomical description of the incision from the xiphisternum to the pubis and from the umbilicus to the mid-axillary line. Fortunately, I had been given epidural anaesthesia as well and my wound did not hurt! I remembered the first thing I had to do; I started wriggling my toes..."

Dr Seth served in the National Health Service as a GP, GP Tutor for Nottingham University and as a Surgeon at the City Hospital and for the Family Planning Association. His special interests were in bladder cancer, vasectomies and erectile dysfunction. He was elected as the President and Trustee of the Nottingham Med-Chi Society in 2002. He is a past President of Nottinghamshire Medico-Legal Society. He is proud to have served in the National Health Service for over 40 years. Dr Seth was appointed MBE by Her Majesty The Queen in 2007 for services to Rotary International and the community in Nottinghamshire.

Soon after his retirement he developed cancer in his kidney, which had to be removed. A year later it spread to his liver and the inferior vena cava (the main vein in the abdomen). He had major surgery again. The cancer then spread to his lungs, which was excised through keyhole surgery. He is now cancer free. While he was lying down in intensive care unit, recovering, he was aware of the preventable dangers of hospitalisation, and he was determined to give himself the best chance of full recovery. He wished that his fellow patients on either side of him and in the wards were also aware of the pitfalls of hospitalisation. This would give everyone a chance of good recovery and avoid complications and unnecessary anxiety. This inspired him to write this booklet.

Useful organisations

Action on Hearing Loss
Tel: 0808 808 0123
Textphone: 0808 808 9000
www.actionhearingloss.org.uk

Age UK
Tel: 0800 169 6565
www.ageuk.org.uk

Alzheimer's Society
Tel: 0845 300 0336
www.alzheimers.org.uk

Asthma UK
Tel: 0800 121 6244
www.asthma.org.uk

Bladder and Bowel Foundation
Tel: 0845 345 0165
www.bladderandbowelfoundation.org

British Heart Foundation
Tel: 0300 330 3311
(medical info or support)
www.bhf.org.uk

Carers UK
Tel: 0808 808 7777
www.carersuk.org

Cinnamon Trust
(Practical help with caring for pets)
Tel: 01736 757 900
www.cinnamon.org.uk

Diabetes UK
Tel: 020 7424 1000
www.diabetes.org.uk

Directgov Health and Wellbeing
www.direct.gov.uk/en/
healthandwellbeing

European Health Insurance Card
Tel: 0845 606 2030
www.ehic.org.uk

Macmillan Cancer Support
Tel: 0808 808 0000
www.macmillan.org.uk

Multiple Sclerosis Society
Tel: 0808 800 8000
www.mssociety.org.uk

NHS Choices Live Well
www.nhs.uk/livewwell

NHS Direct
Tel: 0845 4647
www.nhsdirect.nhs.uk

PALS (Patient Advice and Liaison Service)
Tel: Visit the website to find your local PALS office:
www.pals.nhs.uk

The Patients Association
Tel: 0845 608 4455
www.patients-association.com

RNIB
Tel: 0303 123 9999
www.rnib.org.uk

The Samaritans
Tel: 08457 90 90 90
www.samaritans.org

Stroke Association
Tel: 0303 303 3100
www.stroke.org.uk